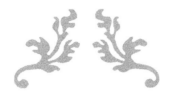

Wood Pellet Smoker And Grill For Beginners

The Succinct Guide Delicious Recipes To Enjoy With Your Family And Friends. Let's Discover All The Techniques And Secrets To Prepare Tasty Dishes For All The Occasions

LIAM JONES

Table of Contents

BREAKFAST RECIPES

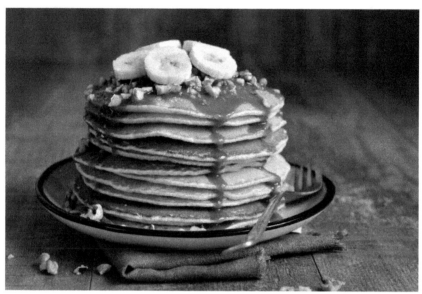

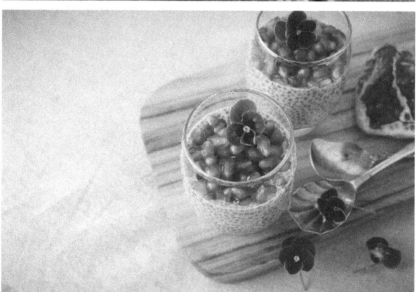

1. *Ice Cream Bread*

Preparation Time: 10 minutes

Cooking Time: 1 hour

Servings: 6

Ingredients:

- 1 ½ quart full-fat butter pecan ice cream, softened
- 1 teaspoon salt
- 2 cups semisweet chocolate chips
- 1 cup sugar
- 1 stick melted butter
- Butter, for greasing
- 4 cups self-rising flour

Directions:

1. Add wood pellets to your smoker and follow your cooker's startup procedure. Preheat your smoker, with your lid closed, until it reaches 350.
2. Mix the salt, sugar, flour, and ice cream with an electric mixer set to medium for two minutes.
3. As the mixer is still running, add in the chocolate chips, beating until everything is blended.

4. Spray a Bundt pan or tube pan with cooking spray. If you choose to use a solid plan, the center will take too long to cook. That's why a tube or Bundt pan works best.

5. Add the batter to your prepared pan.

6. Set the cake on the grill, cover, and smoke for 50 minutes to an hour. A toothpick should come out clean.

7. Take the pan off of the grill. For 10 minutes cool the bread. Remove carefully the bread from the pan and then drizzle it with some melted butter.

Nutrition: Calories: 148.7 Protein: 3.5g Carbs: 27g Fat: 3g

2. *Grilled Pound Cake with Fruit Dressing*

Preparation Time: 20 Minutes

Cooking Time: 50 Minutes

Servings: 12

Ingredients:

- 1buttermilk pound cake, sliced into 3/4-inch slices
- 1/8 cup butter, melted
- 1.1/2 cup whipped cream
- 1/2 cup blueberries
- 1/2 cup raspberries
- 1/2 cup strawberries, sliced

Directions:

1. Preheat pellet grill to 400°F. Turn your smoke setting too high, if applicable.
2. Brush both sides of each pound cake slice with melted butter.
3. Place directly on the grill grate and cook for 5 minutes per side. Turn 90° halfway through cooking each side of the cake for checkered grill marks.
4. You can cook a couple of minutes longer if you prefer deeper grill marks and smoky flavor.
5. Remove pound cake slices from the grill and allow them to cool on a plate.

6. Top the slices with whipped cream, blueberries, raspberries, and sliced strawberries as desired. Serve and enjoy!

Nutrition: Calories: 222.1 Fat: 8.7 g Cholesterol: 64.7 mg Carbohydrate: 33.1 g Fiber: 0.4 g Sugar: 20.6 g Protein: 3.4 g

3. *Grilled Pineapple with Chocolate Sauce*

Preparation Time: 10 Minutes

Cooking Time: 25 Minutes

Servings: 8

Ingredients:

- 1pineapple
- 8 oz bittersweet chocolate chips
- 1/2 cup spiced rum
- 1/2 cup whipping cream
- 2tbsp light brown sugar

Directions:

1. Preheat pellet grill to 400°F.
2. De-skin the pineapple, then slice the pineapple into 1 in cubes.
3. In a saucepan, combine chocolate chips. When chips begin to melt, add rum to the saucepan. Continue to stir until combined, then add a splash of the pineapple's juice.
4. Add in whipping cream and continue to stir the mixture. Once the sauce is smooth and thickening, lower heat to simmer to keep warm.
5. Thread pineapple cubes onto skewers. Sprinkle skewers with brown sugar.

6. Place skewers on the grill grate. Grill for about 5 minutes per side, or until grill marks begin to develop.

7. Remove skewers from the grill and allow to rest on a plate for about 5 minutes. Serve alongside warm chocolate sauce for dipping.

Nutrition: Calories: 112.6 Fat: 0.5 g Cholesterol: 0 Carbohydrate: 28.8 g Fiber: 1.6 g Sugar: 0.1 g Protein: 0.4 g

4. *Nectarine and Nutella Sundae*

Preparation Time: 10 Minutes

Cooking Time: 25 Minutes

Servings: 4

Ingredients:

- 2nectarines halved and pitted
- 2tsp honey
- 4tbsp Nutella
- 4scoops vanilla ice cream
- 1/4 cup pecans, chopped
- Whipped cream, to top
- 4cherries, to top

Directions:

1. Preheat pellet grill to 400°F.
2. Slice nectarines in half and remove the pits.
3. Brush the inside (cut side) of each nectarine half with honey.
4. Place nectarines directly on the grill grate, cut side down—Cook for 5-6 minutes, or until grill marks develop.
5. Flip nectarines and cook on the other side for about 2 minutes.
6. Remove nectarines from the grill and allow it to cool.
7. Fill the pit cavity on each nectarine half with 1 tbsp Nutella.

8. Place one scoop of ice cream on top of Nutella. Top with whipped cream, cherries, and sprinkle chopped pecans. Serve and enjoy!

Nutrition: Calories: 90 Fat: 3 g Carbohydrate: 15g Sugar: 13 g Protein: 2 g

FISH AND SEAFOOD RECIPES

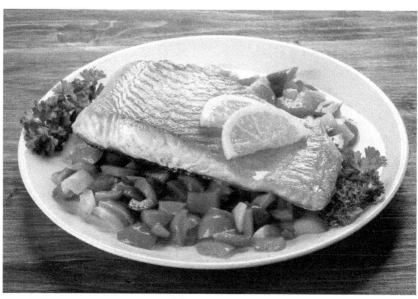

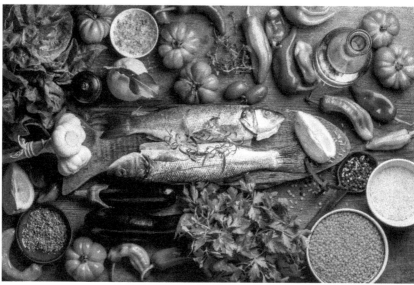

5. *Salmon Burgers*

Preparation Time: 5 Minutes

Cooking Time: 11 Minutes

Servings: 4

Ingredients:

- 1½ pounds salmon fillet, skin, and any remaining pin bones removed, cut into chunks
- 2 teaspoons Dijon mustard
- 3 scallions, trimmed and chopped
- ¼ cup bread crumbs (preferably fresh)
- Salt and pepper
- Good-quality olive oil for brushing
- sesame hamburger buns or 8–10 slider buns (like potato or dinner rolls)
- 1 large tomato, cut into 4 thick slices

Directions:

1. Put about one-quarter of the salmon and the mustard in a food processor and purée into a paste. Add the rest of the salmon and pulse until chopped. Transfer to a bowl, add the scallions, bread crumbs, and a sprinkle of salt and pepper. Mix gently just enough to combine. Form into 4 burgers ¾ to 1

inch thick. Transfer to a plate, cover with plastic wrap and chill until firm, at least 2 or up to 8 hours.

2. Turn the control knob to the high position, when the pellet grill is hot, brush the burgers with oil on both sides, then put them on the pellet grill. Cook for 11 minutes.

3. After 11 minutes, check the burgers for doneness. Cooking is complete when the internal temperature reaches at least 165°F on a food thermometer. If necessary, close the hood and continue cooking for up to 2 minutes more.

4. Remove the burgers from the pellet grill.

5. Put the buns on the pellet grill, cut side down, and toast for 1 to 2 minutes. Serve the burgers on the buns, topped with the tomato if using.

Nutrition: Calories: 123; Fat: 21g; Protein:16g; Fiber:12g

6. *Basil-Ginger Shrimp Burgers*

Preparation Time: 5 Minutes

Cooking Time: 10 Minutes

Servings: 4

Ingredients:

- large clove garlic, peeled
- 1 1-inch piece fresh ginger, peeled and
- sliced
- 1½ pounds shrimp, peeled (and deveined if you like)
- ½ cup lightly packed fresh basil leaves
- ¼ cup roughly chopped shallots, scallions, or red onion
- Salt and pepper
- Sesame oil for brushing the burgers
- sesame hamburger buns or 8–10 slider buns
- Lime wedges for serving
- Lettuce, sliced tomato, and other
- condiments for serving (optional)

Directions:

1. Put the garlic, ginger, and one-third of the shrimp in a food processor; purée until smooth, stopping the machine to scrape down the sides as necessary. Add the remaining shrimp, basil, and shallots, season with salt and pepper, and

pulse to chop. Form into 4 burgers about ¾ inch thick (or 8 to 10 sliders). Transfer to a plate, cover with plastic wrap and chill until firm, at least 1 or up to 8 hours.

2. Turn the control knob to the high position, when the pellet grill is hot, brush the burgers on both sides with oil then put them on the pellet grill and cook until the bottoms brown and they release easily, 5 to 7 minutes. Carefully turn and cook until opaque all the way through, 3 to 5 minutes. Put the buns, cut side down, on the pellet grill to toast. Serve the burgers on the toasted buns with lime wedges, as is or dressed however you like.

Nutrition: Calories: 194; Fat: 21g; Protein:6g; Fiber:2g

7. *Perfectly Smoked Turkey Legs*

Preparation Time: 15 Minutes

Cooking Time: 4 Hours

Servings: 6

Ingredients:

For Turkey:

- 3 tbsp. Worcestershire sauce
- 1 tbsp. canola oil
- 6 turkey legs

For Rub:

- ¼ C. chipotle seasoning
- 1 tbsp. brown sugar
- 1 tbsp. paprika

For Sauce:

- 1 C. white vinegar
- 1 tbsp. canola oil
- 1 tbsp. chipotle BBQ sauce

Directions:

1. For turkey in a bowl, add the Worcestershire sauce and canola oil and mix well.
2. With your fingers, loosen the skin of your legs.
3. With your fingers coat the legs under the skin with an oil mixture.
4. In another bowl, mix rub ingredients.
5. Rub the spice mixture under and the outer surface of turkey legs generously.
6. Transfer the legs into a large sealable bag and refrigerate for about 2-4 hours.
7. Remove the turkey legs from the refrigerator and set them aside at room temperature for at least 30 mins before cooking.
8. Set the temperature of Wood pellet Grill to 200-220 degrees F and preheat with a closed lid for 15 mins.
9. In a small pan, mix all sauce ingredients on low heat and cook until warmed completely, stirring continuously.
10. Place the turkey legs onto the grill cook for about 3½-4 hours, coating with sauce after every 45 mins.
11. Serve hot.

Nutrition: Calories per serving: 430 Carbohydrates: 4.9g Protein: 51.2g Fat: 19.5g Sugar: 3.9g Sodium: 1474mg Fiber: 0.5g

8. *Authentic Holiday Turkey Breast*

Preparation Time: 15 Minutes

Cooking Time: 4 Hours

Servings: 6

Ingredients:

- ½ C. honey
- ¼ C. dry sherry
- 1 tbsp. butter
- 2 tbsp. fresh lemon juice
- Salt, to taste
- 1 (3-3½-pound) skinless, boneless turkey breast

1. Place honey, sherry, and butter over low heat and cook until the mixture becomes smooth, stirring continuously in a small pan.
2. Remove from heat and stir in lemon juice and salt. Set aside to cool.
3. **Directions**:
4. Transfer the honey mixture and turkey breast to a sealable bag.
5. Seal the bag and shake to coat well.
6. Refrigerate for about 6-10 hours.
7. Set the temperature of Wood pellet Grill to 225-250 degrees F and preheat with a closed lid for 15 mins.

8. Place the turkey breast onto the grill and cook for about 2½-4 hours or until the desired doneness.

9. Remove turkey breast from grill and place onto a cutting board for about 15-20 mins before slicing.

10. With a sharp knife, cut the turkey breast into desired-sized slices and serve.

Nutrition: Calories per serving: 443 Carbohydrates: 23.7g Protein: 59.2g Fat: 11.4g Sugar: 23.4g

Sodium: 138mg Fiber: 0.1g

9. *Succulent Duck Breast*

Preparation Time: 10 Minutes

Cooking Time: 10 Minutes

Servings: 4

Ingredients:

- 4 (6-oz.) boneless duck breasts
- 2 tbsp. chicken rub

Directions:

1. Set the temperature of Wood pellet Grill to 275 degrees F and preheat with a closed lid for 15 mins.
2. With a sharp knife, score the skin of the duck into a ¼-inch diamond pattern.
3. Season the duck breast with rub evenly.
4. Place the duck breasts onto the grill, meat side down, and cook for about 10 mins.
5. Now, set the temperature of Wood pellet Grill to 400 degrees F.
6. Now, arrange the breasts, skin side down, and cook for about 10 mins, flipping once halfway through.
7. Remove from the grill and serve.

Nutrition: Calories per serving: 231 Carbohydrates: 1.5g Protein: 37.4g Fat: 6.8g Sugar: 0g Sodium: 233mg Fiber: 0g

10. *Grilled Chicken Fajitas*

Preparation Time: 30 Minutes

Cooking Time: 45 Minutes

Servings: 4

Ingredients:

- 1 lb. boneless skinless chicken breast
- 1/2 green bell pepper, julienned
- 8 tortillas, flour, or corn
- 1/2 red bell pepper, julienned
- 1 avocado, sliced
- Toppings: shredded cheese, salsa,
- 1/2 cup yellow onion, julienned
- guacamole, sour cream, jalapeños

RUB INGREDIENTS

- 1 tsp kosher salt
- 1 tsp garlic powder
- 1 tsp dried oregano
- 1 tsp chili powder
- 1 tsp cumin
- 1 tsp paprika

Directions:

1. Preheat your pellet grill to 350°F.
2. Mix all rub ingredients in a small bowl.
3. Rinse chicken underwater then coat the chicken with the rub mixture, and thoroughly coat the chicken breast.
4. Place chicken breast on the pellet grill and cook, flipping after about 5 minutes. Cook for about 10-12 minutes total, or until no longer pink.
5. After chicken has cooked all the way through, put out from heat and allow to rest for 10 minutes.
6. Add onions, green pepper, and red pepper to a stove pan in your kitchen while the chicken rests. Add a splash of olive oil (if desired) and sauté the veggies for about 8 minutes or until they begin to soften.
7. Slice the chicken into thin strips.
8. Serve immediately on corn or flour tortillas. Add onions and avocado slices.
9. Squeeze lime wedges over the steak and add any additional toppings as desired like shredded cheese, salsa, guacamole, sour cream, etc.

Nutrition: Calories per serving: 430 Carbohydrates: 2.1g Protein: 25.4g Fat: 33g Sodium: 331mg Fiber: 0.7g

11. *Pellet Grill Beer Can Chicken*

Preparation Time: 10 Minutes

Cooking Time: 2 Hours and 15 Minutes

Servings: 4 to 6

Ingredients:

- 1 whole chicken (3-5 lbs.)
- 1 tbsp ground black pepper
- 2 tbsp paprika
- 2 tsp dried thyme
- 2 tbsp kosher salt
- 2 tsp dried oregano
- 2 tbsp onion powder
- 2 tsp garlic powder
- 1 tbsp cayenne pepper
- Vegetable oil, to lightly coat chicken
- 1 tbsp ground cumin
- 1 can beer (12 oz)

Directions:

1. Preheat pellet grill to 350°F.
2. Lightly brush chicken with a thin layer of vegetable oil.
3. Mix all other seasoning ingredients in a small bowl.

4. Rub the chicken down thoroughly with seasoning mixture, ensuring to season the cavity.

5. Open beer can and pour out (or drink) 1/4 of the beer. The place opened a beer can in the chicken's cavity, with the bottom of the can sticking out.

6. Place chicken on a sheet tray with raised edges. You can also utilize a beer can chicken roaster rack instead of a sheet tray. Place sheet tray with chicken onto the center of the cooking grate and cook for approximately 2 hours.

7. The chicken is done once it reaches an internal temperature of 165°F in the breast's centermost point, regardless of how long it has been on the grill.

8. Allow resting for 10 minutes. Carve, serve, and enjoy!

Nutrition: Calories per serving: 430 Carbohydrates: 2.1g Protein: 25.4g Fat: 33g Sodium: 331mg Fiber: 0.7g

12. *Grilled Club Chicken Lettuce Wraps*

Preparation Time: 20 Minutes

Cooking Time: 45 Minutes

Servings: 4

Ingredients:

- 1 1/2 lb. boneless skinless chicken breast
- 1 avocado, sliced
- 1/2 tbsp ground black pepper
- 4 slices cooked thick-cut bacon, chopped
- 1/2 tbsp kosher salt
- 8 large iceberg lettuce leaves
- 1 cup grape tomatoes, diced
- Ranch dressing

Directions:

1. Preheat your pellet grill to 350°F.
2. Mix fresh ground pepper and kosher salt in a small bowl.
3. Season chicken breast with salt and pepper mixture.
4. Place chicken breast on the pellet grill and cook until no longer pink, flipping after about 5 minutes.
5. After the chicken has cooked, remove it from heat and allow to rest for 10 minutes.
6. Slice chicken breast into thin strips.

7. Divide chicken among the 8 large iceberg lettuce leaves. Top with diced tomatoes, avocado, diced bacon, and drizzle with ranch dressing. Serve and enjoy!

Nutrition: Calories per serving: 430 Carbohydrates: 2.1g Protein: 25.4g Fat: 33g Sodium: 331mg Fiber: 0.7g

13. _Hot and Spicy Grilled Chicken Wings_

Preparation Time: 15 Minutes

Cooking Time: 45 Minutes

Servings: 4

Ingredients:

- 4 lbs. chicken wings
- Sauce ingredients
- 1/2 cup ketchup
- tbsp yellow onion, minced
- 1/4 cup water
- 1 tbsp Worcestershire sauce
- 1/4 cup honey
- 1 tbsp soy sauce
- 1/4 cup white vinegar
- 2 tbsp hot sauce
- 2 tbsp light brown sugar
- 3 cloves garlic, minced

Directions:

1. Preheat your pellet grill to 400°F.
2. In a saucepan, blend all sauce ingredients and bring to a boil over medium heat. Then, reduce heat and simmer for 15

minutes. During this time, sample the sauce and determine if it's the right level of spicy for you. Add hot sauce as needed.

3. Add wings to a separate, large bowl. Pour sauce over wings in the bowl. Toss wings to completely and thoroughly coat with sauce.

4. Place wings on cookie sheet and transfer to grill. Place wings on grill grate and cook for 30 minutes, flipping halfway through after 15 minutes.

5. Remove wings from grill after they are thoroughly cooked and crispy on the outside.

6. Allow to cool at room temperature for 10 minutes then serve and enjoy!

Nutrition: Calories per serving: 430 Carbohydrates: 2.1g Protein: 25.4g Fat: 33g Sodium: 331mg Fiber: 0.7g

BEEF RECIPES

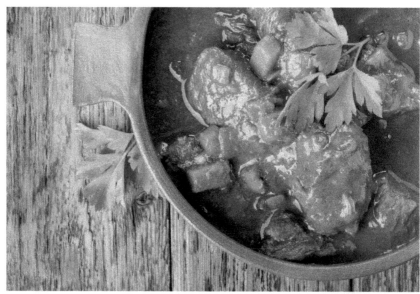

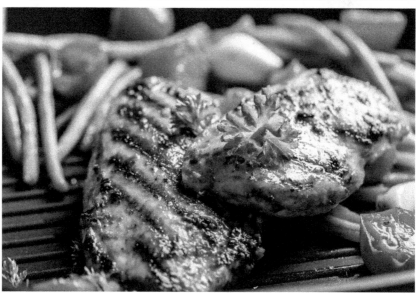

14. *Smoked Italian Meatballs*

Preparation Time: 10 minutes

Cooking Time: 30 minutes

Servings: 8

Ingredients:

- 1-pound ground beef
- 1-pound Italian Sausage
- ½ cup Italian breadcrumbs
- 1 teaspoon dry mustard
- ½ cup parmesan cheese (grated)
- 1 teaspoon Italian seasoning
- 1 jalapeno (finely chopped)
- 2 eggs
- 1 teaspoon salt
- 1 onion (finely chopped)
- 2 teaspoon garlic powder
- ½ teaspoon smoked paprika
- 1 teaspoon oregano
- 1 teaspoon crushed red pepper
- 1 tablespoon Worcestershire sauce

Directions:

1. Combine all the ingredients in a large mixing bowl. Mix until the ingredients are well combined.
2. Mold the mixture into 1 ½ inch balls and arrange the balls into a greased baking sheet.
3. Preheat the wood pellet smoker to 180°F, using a hickory pellet.
4. Arrange the meatballs on the grill and smoke for 20 minutes.
5. Increase the griller's temperature to 350°F and smoke until the internal temperature of the meatballs reaches 165°F.
6. Remove the meatballs from the grill and let them cool for a few minutes.
7. Serve warm and enjoy.

Nutrition: Carbohydrates: 12g | Protein: 28g | Fat: 16g | Sodium: 23mg Cholesterol: 21mg

15. *Braised Short Ribs*

Preparation Time: 25 minutes

Cooking Time: 4 hours

Servings: 2 to 4

Ingredients:

- 4 beef short ribs
- Salt
- Freshly ground black pepper
- ½ cup beef broth

Directions:

1. Supply your smoker with wood pellets and follow the manufacturer's specific start-up procedure. With the lid closed, let the grill heat to 180°F.
2. Season the ribs on both sides with salt and pepper.
3. Place the ribs directly on the grill grate and smoke for 3 hours.
4. Pull the ribs from the grill and place them on enough aluminum foil to wrap them completely.
5. Increase the grill's temperature to 375°F.
6. Fold in three sides of the foil around the ribs and add the beef broth. Fold in the last side, completely enclosing the ribs and liquid.
7. Return the wrapped ribs to the grill and cook for 45 minutes more.

8. Remove the short ribs from the grill, unwrap them, and serve immediately.

9. Master Tip:

10. Adding herbs to your wraps, such as rosemary or thyme, can contribute some fresh, delicious flavor to the short ribs.

Nutrition: Calories: 240 | Fat: 23g Carbohydrates: 1g Dietary Fiber 0g | Protein: 33g

16. Perfect Roast Prime Ribs

Preparation Time: 15 minutes

Cooking Time: 4 or 5 hours

Servings: 4 to 6

Ingredients:

- 1 (3-bone) rib roast
- Salt
- Freshly ground black pepper
- 1 garlic clove, minced

Directions:

1. Supply your smoker with wood pellets and follow the manufacturer's specific start-up procedure. With the lid closed, let the grill heat to 360°F.

2. Season the roast all over with salt and pepper and, with the use of your hands, rub it all over with the minced garlic.

3. Place the roast directly on the grill grate and smoke for 4 or 5 hours, until its internal temperature reaches 145°F for medium-rare.

4. Take the roast off the grill and let it rest for 15 minutes, before slicing and serving.

Nutrition: Calories: 250 | Fat: 25g Carbohydrates: 3g Dietary Fiber: 0g | Protein: 40g Master Tip: This same recipe can be used for a 5- or 7-bone rib roast. Just increase the smoking time and the garlic, as desired.

17. Smoked Lamb Leg

Preparation Time: 30 minutes

Cooking Time: 3 hours

Servings: 6

Ingredients

- 6 cloves garlic

- 1 lb. tomatillos

- 1 onion

- 5 chili peppers

- 1 tablespoon capers

- 1/4 cup cilantro

- 1/2 teaspoon sugar

- Salt and pepper

- 2 tablespoons olive oil

- 1 cup chicken broth

- 3 tablespoons lime juice

- 1 leg of lamb

- 2 tablespoon rosemary

Directions:

1. When ready to cook, set your smoker to 450 deg and preheat. Skewer the tomatillos, onions, and chilis, then grill for nine minutes.

2. Take all of that off the grill and place a large pan on the grill. Blend the earlier skewered vegetables, adding sugar and cilantro.

3. Add oil to the pan, followed by the mixture. Add the chicken broth and lime juice and reduce for 20 minutes. Take out and chill, then set your smoker to 180 deg.

4. Slice into the lamb and stuff the gaps with garlic before seasoning with salt, rosemary, and pepper. Smoke the lamb for 30 minutes.

5. Increase the temperature to 350 deg and cook for another two hours.

6. Take out and let stand before serving with your salsa verde.

Nutrition: Calories 390, Total fat 35g, Saturated fat 15g, Total Carbs 0g, Net Carbs 0g, Protein 17g, Sugar 0g, Fiber 0g, Sodium: 65mg.

18. Lamb Rack

Preparation Time: 10 minutes

Cooking Time: 30 minutes

Servings: 4

Ingredients

- 8 cloves garlic
- 1 bunch fresh thyme
- 1 tablespoon salt
- 2 teaspoons olive oil
- 1 teaspoon sherry vinegar
- 2 lbs. rack of lamb

Directions:

1. Blend the garlic and thyme with salt, vinegar, and oil. Rub the mix over the rack of lamb.
2. When ready to cook, set your smoker to 450 deg and preheat.
3. Grill the lamb for 20 minutes' fat-side down. Turn and grill for ten more minutes before slicing and serving.

Nutrition: Calories 390, Total fat 35g, Saturated fat 15g, Total Carbs 0g, Net Carbs 0g, Protein 17g, Sugar 0g, Fiber 0g, Sodium: 65mg.

19. Barqued Leg of Lamb

Preparation Time 30 Mins

Cooking Time 90 Mins

Servings 8-12

Ingredients:

- 1 (7-8 lb.) leg of lamb, bone-in
- 1 tbsp garlic, crushed
- 4 cloves garlic, sliced lengthwise
- 4 sprigs rosemary, cut into 1" pieces
- 2 tsp olive oil
- 2 lemons
- Salt and pepper, to taste

Directions:

1. Combine olive oil and crushed garlic. Rub the mixture on the leg of lamb.

2. With a paring knife, make small 3/4-inch deep perforations in the lamb, about 2 dozen. Stuff the slivered garlic and cut rosemary sprigs into the perforations.

3. Zest and juice the lemons, spreading the zest and juice evenly over the lamb. Season lamb with salt and pepper.

4. When ready to cook, set temperature to High and preheat, lid closed for 15 minutes.

5. Place the leg of lamb on the grill and cook for 30 minutes.

6. Reduce grill temperature to 350°F and cook until the internal temperature reaches 130°F for medium-rare, about 60-90 minutes.

7. Let the lamb rest for 15 minutes before carving. Enjoy!

Nutrition: Calories 390, Total fat 35g, Saturated fat 15g, Total Carbs 0g, Net Carbs 0g, Protein 17g, Sugar 0g, Fiber 0g, Sodium: 65mg.

PORK RECIPES

20. *Wood Pellet Pulled Pork*

Preparation Time: 15 Minutes

Cooking Time: 12 Hours

Servings: 12

Ingredients:

- 8 lb. pork shoulder roast, bone-in
- BBQ rub
- 3 cups apple cider, dry hard

Directions:

1. Fire up the wood pellet grill and set it to smoke.
2. Meanwhile, rub the pork with BBQ rub on all sides, then place it on the grill grates. Cook for 5 hours, flipping it every 1 hour.
3. Increase the heat to 225°F and continue cooking for 3 hours directly on the grate.
4. Transfer the pork to a foil pan and place the apple cider at the bottom of the pan.
5. Cook until the internal temperature reaches 200°F then remove it from the grill. Wrap the pork loosely with foil, then let it rest for 1 hour.
6. Remove the fat layer and use forks to shred it.

7. Serve and enjoy.

Nutrition: Calories 912 Total fat 65g Saturated fat 24g Total Carbs 7g Net Carbs 7g Protein 70g Sugar 6g

0g Sodium: 208mg

21. Lovable Pork Belly

Preparation Time: 15 Minutes

Cooking Time: 4 Hours and 30 Minutes

Servings: 4

Ingredients:

- 5 pounds of pork belly
- 1 cup dry rub
- Three tablespoons olive oil

For Sauce

- Two tablespoons honey
- Three tablespoons butter
- 1 cup BBQ sauce

Directions:

1. Take your drip pan and add water. Cover with aluminum foil.
2. Pre-heat your smoker to 250 degrees F
3. Add pork cubes, dry rub, olive oil into a bowl and mix well
4. Use water fill water pan halfway through and place it over drip pan.
5. Add wood chips to the side tray
6. Transfer pork cubes to your smoker and smoke for 3 hours (covered)

7. Remove pork cubes from the smoker and transfer to foil pan, add honey, butter, BBQ sauce, and stir

8. Cover the pan with foil and move back to a smoker, smoke for 90 minutes more

9. Remove foil and smoke for 15 minutes more until the sauce thickens

10. Serve and enjoy!

Nutrition: Calories: 1164 Fat: 68g Carbohydrates: 12g Protein: 104g

22. *County Ribs*

Preparation Time: 15 Minutes

Cooking Time: 3 Hours

Servings: 4

Ingredients:

- 4 pounds country-style ribs
- Pork rub to taste
- 2 cups apple juice
- ½ stick butter, melted
- 18 ounces BBQ sauce

Directions:

1. Take your drip pan and add water. Cover with aluminum foil.
2. Pre-heat your smoker to 275 degrees F
3. Season country style ribs from all sides
4. Use water fill water pan halfway through and place it over drip pan.
5. Add wood chips to the side tray.
6. Transfer the ribs to your smoker and smoke for 1 hour and 15 minutes until the internal temperature reaches 160 degrees F
7. Take foil pan and mix melted butter, apple juice, 15 ounces BBQ sauce and put ribs back in the pan, cover with foil

8. Transfer back to smoker and smoke for 1 hour 15 minutes more until the internal temperature reaches 195 degrees F

9. Take ribs out from liquid and place them on racks, glaze ribs with more BBQ sauce, and smoke for 10 minutes more

10. Take them out and let them rest for 10 minutes, serve and enjoy!

Nutrition: Calories: 251 Fat: 25g Carbohydrates: 35g Protein: 76g

23. Wow-Pork Tenderloin

Preparation Time: 15 Minutes

Cooking Time: 3 Hours

Servings: 4

Ingredients:

- One pork tenderloin
- ¼ cup BBQ sauce
- Three tablespoons dry rub

Directions:

1. Take your drip pan and add water. Cover with aluminum foil.
2. Pre-heat your smoker to 225 degrees F
3. Rub the spice mix all over the pork tenderloin
4. Use water fill water pan halfway through and place it over drip pan.
5. Add wood chips to the side tray
6. Transfer pork meat to your smoker and smoke for 3 hours until the internal temperature reaches 145 degrees F
7. Brush the BBQ sauce over pork and let it rest
8. Serve and enjoy!

Nutrition: Calories: 405 Fat: 9g Carbohydrates: 15g Protein: 59g

24. *Carolina Smoked Ribs*

Preparation Time: 30 Minutes

Cooking Time: 4 Hours and 30 Minutes

Servings: 10

Ingredients:

- 1/2 a cup of brown sugar
- 1/3 cup of fresh lemon juice
- ¼ cup of white vinegar
- 1/4 cup of apple cider vinegar
- One tablespoon of Worcestershire sauce
- ¼ cup of molasses
- 2 cups of prepared mustard
- Two teaspoons of garlic, minced
- Two teaspoons of salt
- One teaspoon of ground black pepper
- One teaspoon of crushed red pepper flakes
- ½ a teaspoon of white pepper
- ¼ teaspoon of cayenne pepper
- Two racks of pork spare ribs
- ½ a cup of barbeque seasoning

Directions:

1. Take a medium-sized bowl and whisk in brown sugar, white vinegar, lemon juice, mustard, Worcestershire sauce, mustard, molasses

2. Mix well and season the mixture with granulated garlic, pepper, salt, red pepper flakes, white pepper flakes, cayenne pepper

3. Take your drip pan and add water; cover with aluminum foil.

4. Pre-heat your smoker to 225 degrees F

5. Use water fill water pan halfway through and place it over drip pan.

6. Add wood chips to the side tray

7. Rub the ribs with your prepared seasoning and transfer to your smoker

8. Cover the meat with aluminum foil and smoke for 4 hours, making sure to add chips after every 60 minutes

9. After the first three and a ½ hours, make sure to uncover the meat and baste it generously with the prepared mustard sauce

10. Take the heart out and serve with the remaining sauce

11. Enjoy!

Nutrition: Calories: 750 Fat: 50g Carbohydrates: 24g Fiber: 2.2g

25. *Premium Sausage Hash*

Preparation Time: 30 Minutes

Cooking Time: 45 Minutes

Servings: 4

Ingredients:

- Nonstick cooking spray
- Two finely minced garlic cloves
- One teaspoon basil, dried
- One teaspoon oregano, dried
- One teaspoon onion powder
- One teaspoon of salt
- 4-6 cooked smoker Italian Sausage (Sliced)
- One large-sized bell pepper, diced
- One large onion, diced
- Three potatoes, cut into 1-inch cubes
- Three tablespoons of olive oil
- French bread for serving

Directions:

1. Pre-heat your smoker to 225 degrees Fahrenheit using your desired wood chips

2. Cover the smoker grill rack with foil and coat with cooking spray

3. Take a small bowl and add garlic, oregano, basil, onion powder, and season the mix with salt and pepper
4. Take a large bowl and add sausage slices, bell pepper, potatoes, onion, olive oil, and spice mix
5. Mix well and spread the mixture on your foil-covered rack
6. Place the rack in your smoker and smoke for 45 minutes
7. Serve with your French bread
8. Enjoy!

Nutrition: Calories: 193 Fats: 10g Carbs: 15g Fiber: 2g

APPETIZERS AND SIDES

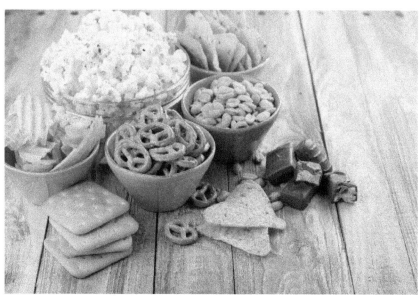

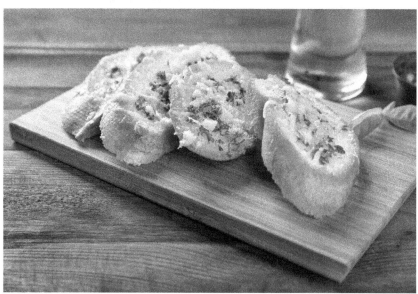

26. *Mesmerizing Banana Foster*

Preparation Time: 10-15 minutes

Cooking Time: 15-20 minutes

Servings: 4

Ingredients

- 10 bananas, overripe, peeled, and halved lengthwise
- Rum and raisin sauce for serving

Directions:

1. Take your drip pan and add water, cover with aluminum foil. Pre-heat your smoker to 250 degrees F
2. Use water fill water pan halfway through and place it over drip pan. Add wood chips to the side tray
3. Take a large-sized disposable aluminum foil, arrange bananas in a single layer
4. Transfer to smoker and smoke for 15-20 minutes
5. Serve with rum and raisin sauce, enjoy!

Nutrition: Calories: 355 Fat: 12g Carbohydrates: 41g Protein: 1g

27. Stuffed Up Chorizo Pepper

Preparation Time: 10-15 minutes

Cooking Time: 2 hours

Servings: 4

Ingredients

- 3 cups cheese, shredded

- 2 pounds chorizo, ground

- 4 poblano pepper, halved and seeded

- 8 bacon slices, uncooked

Directions:

1. Take your drip pan and add water, cover with aluminum foil. Pre-heat your smoker to 225 degrees F

2. Use water fill water pan halfway through and place it over drip pan. Add wood chips to the side tray

3. Divide the mix into 8 portions and press one portion into each pepper half

4. Sprinkle the rest of the cheddar on top

5. Wrap each pepper half with 1 bacon slice, making sure to tuck in the edges to secure it

6. Transfer peppers to your smoker and smoke for 2 hours until the internal temperature of the sausage reach 165-degree Fahrenheit

7. Enjoy!

Nutrition: Calories: 834 Fats: 51g Carbs: 55g Fiber: 2g

28. Cool Brie Cheese

Preparation Time: 10-15 minutes

Cooking Time: 60 minutes

Servings: 4

Ingredients

8-ounce blocks of brie cheese

Directions:

- Take your drip pan and add water, cover with aluminum foil. Pre-heat your smoker to 90 degrees Flow settings
- Use water fill water pan halfway through and place it over drip pan. Add wood chips to the side tray
- Add cheese blocks to your smoker and let them smoke for 4 hours
- Remove from heat and let them cool at room temperature
- Transfer to a container, serve, and enjoy!

Nutrition: Calories: 100 Fat: 9g Carbohydrates: 0g Protein: 4g

29. *Spectacular Smoked Peach*

Preparation Time: 20 minutes

Cooking Time: 35-45 minutes

Servings: 4

Ingredients

- tablespoons honey
- 1-pint vanilla ice cream
- 1 tablespoon packed brown sugar
- 4 barely ripe peaches, halved and 3 pitted

Directions:

1. Take your drip pan and add water, cover with aluminum foil. Pre-heat your smoker to 200 degrees F
2. Use water fill water pan halfway through and place it over drip pan. Add wood chips to the side tray
3. Sprinkle cut peach halves with brown sugar
4. Transfer prepared peach to smoker and smoke for 30-45 minutes
5. Drizzle honey and serve
6. Enjoy!

Nutrition: Calories: 309 Fats: 27g Carbs: 17g Fiber: 2g

30. Meaty Bologna

Preparation Time: 20 minutes

Cooking Time:60 minutes

Serving: 6-8

Ingredients

- Salt and pepper to taste
- ¼ cup yellow mustard
- 5 pounds all-beef bologna chub
- 1 teaspoon garlic powder
- 1 teaspoon ground nutmeg
- 1 teaspoon ground coriander
- 2 tablespoons packed brown sugar
- 2 tablespoons chili powder

Directions:

1. Take your drip pan and add water, cover with aluminum foil. Pre-heat your smoker to 250 degrees F
2. Use water fill water pan halfway through and place it over drip pan. Add wood chips to the side tray
3. Take a small-sized bowl and add chili powder, coriander, nutmeg, brown sugar, garlic
4. Mix well and keep it on the side

5. Cut bologna into ½ inch slices, making sure that there are few small cuts all around the edges

6. Coat them generously with mustard mix

7. Season generously with salt and pepper, spice mix

8. Transfer to Smoker and smoke for 1 hour

9. Serve and enjoy once done!

Nutrition: Calories: 819 Fats: 46g Carbs: 1g Fiber: 2g

31. *Simple Dump Cake*

Preparation Time: 20 minutes

Cooking Time: 60 – 120 minutes

Servings: 6-8

Ingredients

- 1 box cake mix of your choosing
- 2 cans of your desired pie filling
- 1 stick of butter

Directions:

1. Take your drip pan and add water, cover with aluminum foil. Pre-heat your smoker to 250 degrees F
2. Use water fill water pan halfway through and place it over drip pan. Add wood chips to the side tray
3. Spread the contents of the pie to the bottom of a container, sprinkle cake mix on top
4. Melt butter in a saucepot and drizzle over cake mix
5. Transfer to the smoker and bake for about 60-120 minutes
6. Enjoy!

Nutrition: Calories: 328 Fat: 9g Carbohydrates: 61g Protein: 2g

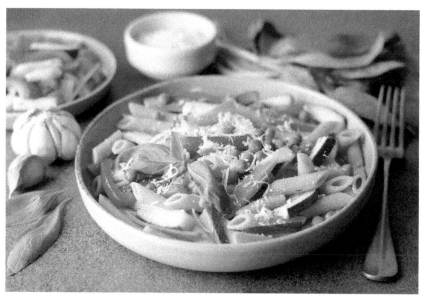

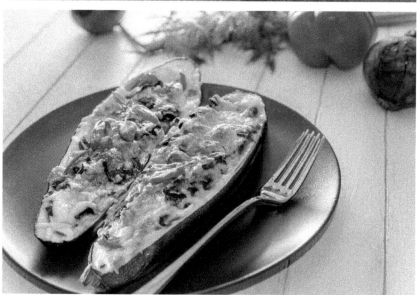

32. *Smoked Broccoli*

Preparation Time: 10 minutes

Cooking Time: 30 minutes

Servings: 4

Ingredients:

- 2 heads broccoli
- Kosher salt
- 2 tablespoons vegetable oil
- Fresh Pepper (ground)

Directions:

1. Preheat your smoker to 350F.
2. Separate the florets from the heads.
3. Coat the broccoli with vegetable oil by tossing. Thereafter, season with salt and pepper.
4. Using a grilling basket, put the broccoli on the grate of the smoker and smoke for 30 minutes or till crisp.
5. Enjoy!

Nutrition: Calories- 76| Fat- 7g| Saturated fat- 1.3g| Protein- 1.3g| Carbohydrates- 3.1g|

33. *Smoked Mushrooms 2*

Preparation Time:10 minutes

Cooking Time: 1 hour

Servings: 4

Ingredients:

- 2 lb. mushrooms (Button or Portabella)
- 2 cups Italian dressing
- Pepper
- Salt

Directions:

1. In a gallon zip lock bag, add in the mushrooms.
2. Pour in the Italian dressing in the zip lock bag and some pepper and salt to taste.
3. Refrigerate for 1 hour.
4. Once ready to cook, preheat your smoker to 250F.
5. Smoke mushrooms for an hour or till much soft and a bit were smaller in size.
6. Note: mushrooms will smoke well at any temperature so long as they don't burn.

Nutrition: Calories- 392| Fat- 34g| Saturated fat- 5.3g| Carbohydrates- 19.8g| Fiber- 2.3g| Sugar- 13.7g| Protein- 7.6g| Cholesterol- 79mg| Sodium- 196mg|

34. *Smoke-Grilled Eggplant*

Preparation Time: 10 minutes

Cooking Time: 10 minutes

Servings: 4

Ingredients:

- 1 eggplant (large in size)
- 4 tablespoons coconut aminos
- 2 tablespoons avocado oil
- 2 teaspoons cumin (ground)
- 2 teaspoons smoked paprika
- 2 teaspoons coriander (ground)
- 2 teaspoons cumin (ground)
- 1/2 teaspoon cayenne pepper
- 1/2 teaspoon garlic powder
- 1/2 teaspoon sea salt

Directions:

1. Cut the eggplant lengthwise to 1/4-inch slices. Drizzle and brush the eggplant slices with coconut aminos and avocado oil.

2. In a small mixing bowl, combine the spices. Sprinkle the mix on the slices on both sides, ensuring they are fully coated.

3. Preheat your grill to medium-high heat and place the slices. Grill each side for 3 minutes till they become tender.

4. Remove from the grill and enjoy.

<u>Nutrition:</u> Calories- 62| Fat- 1.5g| Saturated fat- 0.2g| Carbohydrates- 11.6g| Protein- 1.6g| Calcium- 23mg| Potassium- 337mg| Iron- 1mg|

35. Smoked Cabbage

Preparation Time: 15 minutes

Cooking Time: 1 hour

Servings: 4

Ingredients:

- 1 cabbage
- 1/4 cup olive oil
- Garlic powder
- Black pepper
- Kosher salt

Sauce ingredients:

- 1/4 cup cilantro
- 2 cloves garlic (minced)
- 2 green onions (divided into green parts & white parts)
- Lime juice (2 limes)
- 1 jalapeno (chopped)
- 1 green pear (chopped)
- 2 tablespoons olive oil
- 2 tablespoons buttermilk
- 1 tablespoon mayonnaise
- 1 teaspoon black pepper
- 1 teaspoon sea salt

Directions:

1. Preheat your smoker to 250F

2. Peel off the outer cabbage leaves and use a knife to cut 4 quarters.

3. Coat the 4 quarters with olive oil, seasoning with pepper and salt.

4. Place the cabbage quarters on the tray and smoke with the wedge side up for 20 minutes. Flip the cabbage quarters to one wedge side and smoke for 20 minutes and do the same for the other remaining side, smoking for an additional 20 minutes.

5. Remove the cabbage once well-cooked.

6. Put all sauce ingredients in a blender and process. You can adjust its consistency by adding the liquid ingredients to get your preference.

7. Enjoy!

Nutrition: Calories- 303| Protein- 3g| Fat- 23g| Sat fat- 3g|Carbohydrates- 22g| Sugar- 12g| Fiber- 7g| Sodium- 1236mg| Potassium- 457mg| Calcium- 110mg| Vitamin C- 91.1mg| Vitamin A- 390IU|

36. Smoked Vegetables with Vinaigrette

Preparation Time: 15 minutes

Cooking Time: 4 hours

Servings: 4

Ingredients:

- Zucchini (thickly Sliced)
- Red potatoes (small in size & chopped)
- Red onions (chopped)
- Yellow medium squash (thickly sliced)
- Red pepper (chopped)

Vinaigrette ingredients:

- 1/3 cup olive oil
- 1/4 cup vinegar (balsamic)
- 2 teaspoons Dijon mustard
- Pepper
- Salt

Directions:

1. Add and combine balsamic vinegar, olive oil, Mustard, pepper, and salt in a bowl.
2. In a casserole dish, add all the vegetables and combine. Coat the vegetables with the balsamic vinaigrette by tossing.
3. Preheat your smoker to 225F.

4. Put the dish with the vegetables in the smoker and smoke for 4 hours.

Nutrition: Calories- 225| Fat 17.2g| Saturated fat- 2.5g| Carbohydrates- 16.8g| Protein- 2.8g| Sodium- 196mg| Cholesterol- 0mg| Calcium- 35mg| Potassium- 483mg| Iron- 1mg|

37. *Venison Steaks*

Preparation Time: 10 minutes

Cooking Time: 26 minutes

Servings: 4

Ingredients:

- The Meat:
- 10, 6 ounces Venison steaks
- The Marinade:
- 1-liter Sprite, diet
- 6 ounces game rub
- Other Ingredients:
- 2 pounds asparagus
- The Fire:
- Fill hopper of the grill with 2 pounds of wood pellets, maple flavor, and set the grill according to the user manual.
- Switch on the grill, select the "smoke" setting, shut with the lid, and use the control panel to set the temperature to 250 degrees F.

- Wait for 10 to 15 minutes or until the fire starts in the grill and it reaches the set temperature.

Directions:

1. Before preheating the grill, marinate the venison steaks and for this, take a container, pour in the sprite, and then stir in the game rub.

2. Add venison steaks and then let them marinate in the refrigerator for a minimum of 6 hours.

3. Then remove venison steaks from the marinade and pat dry.

4. When the grill has preheated, place steaks on the grilling rack and let smoke for 8 minutes per side or until the control panel shows the internal temperature of 125 degrees F.

5. When done, remove the steak from the grill and let it rest for 10 minutes.

6. Meanwhile, add asparagus to the grilling rack and cook for 10 minutes, turning halfway.

7. Then cut the steak into slices and serve with asparagus.

Nutrition: Amount per 225 g = 1 serving(s) Energy (calories): 156 kcal Protein: 27.42 g Fat: 2 g Carbohydrates: 8.8 g

38. *Mandarin Glazed Hens*

Preparation Time: 20 minutes

Cooking Time: 40minutes

Servings: 4

Ingredients:

- The Meat:
- 5 Cornish game hens, giblets removed
- The Rub:
- 2 tbsp. Onion powder
- 1 tbsp. Garlic powder
- 1 tbsp. Ginger powder
- 1 tbsp. Salt
- 2 tbsp. Olive oil
- The Stuffing:
- 16 Sprigs of thyme
- 2 Orange, cut into quarters
- The Glaze:
- 1 cup Mandarin glaze
- The Fire:
- According to the user manual, fill the grill's hopper with 2 pounds of wood pellets, mesquite flavor, and set the grill.

- Switch on the grill, select the "smoke" setting, shut with the lid, and use the control panel to set the temperature to 375 degrees F.
- Wait for 10 to 15 minutes or until the fire starts in the grill and it reaches the set temperature.

Directions:

1. In the meantime, prepare hens.
2. Prepare the rub. Take a small bowl, place all of its ingredients in it, and stir until mixed.
3. Stuff each hen's cavity with four thyme sprigs and one wedge of orange, then sprinkle the exterior with the prepared rub.
4. Rub hens with oil and then tie the legs of hens with a kitchen string.
5. When the grill has preheated, place hens on the grilling rack and grill for 20 minutes.
6. Then brush hens with mandarin glaze, continue grilling for 20 minutes and then brush again with mandarin glaze.
7. Serve immediately.

Nutrition: Amount per 187 g = 1 serving(s) Energy (calories): 226 kcal Protein: 25.84 g Fat: 10.98 g Carbohydrates: 4.76 g

39. Cajun Crab Stuffed Shrimp and Jicama Corn Salad

Preparation Time: 20 minutes

Cooking Time: 5 minute

Servings: 4

Ingredients:

- 12 Stuffed shrimp
- 16 oz. Lump crab meat
- 1 medium-size Red onion
- ½ tbsp. Minced garlic Seasoning
- 1 Lime juice
- 1 lime zest
- 2 Jalapeno (optional)
- 16 g Ritz Crackers
- 2 slices Bacon

Directions:

1. Pick cartilage from the crab. Combine ingredients wrap with bacon. Grill till browned.
2. Combine all ingredients and chill Jicama corn salad.
3. Place as many as your shrimp can into each shell and turn to crust side up and grill till done. Soft-shell or soft-shelled

(leave the shell on shrimp). Bag shells. Garnish with Crackers.

4. Serve.

Nutrition: Amount per 191 g = 1 serving(s) Energy (calories): 454 kcal Protein: 47.56 g Fat: 9.31 g

Carbohydrates: 51.17 g

SNACKS

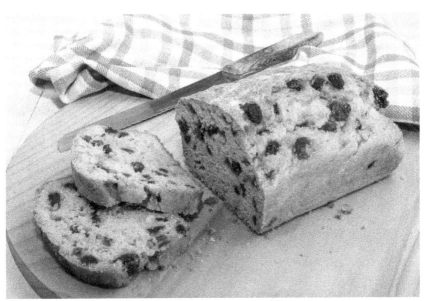

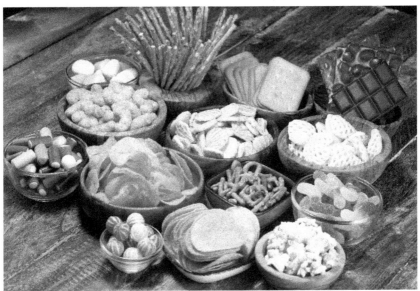

40. Mango Bread

Preparation Time: 15 minutes

Cooking Time: 1 hour

Servings: 4

Ingredients:

- 2 ½ cup cubed ripe mangoes
- 2 cups all-purpose flour
- 1 tsp baking powder
- 1 tsp baking soda
- 2 eggs (beaten)
- 1 tsp cinnamon
- 1 tsp vanilla extract
- ½ tsp nutmeg
- ¾ cup olive oil
- ¾ cup of sugar
- 1 tbsp lemon juice
- ½ tsp salt
- ½ cup chopped dates

Directions:

1. Start your grill on smoke mode and leave the lip opened for 5 minutes, or until the fire starts.

2. Close the lid and preheat the grill to 350°F for 15 minutes, using alder hardwood pellets.

3. Grease an 8 by 4-inch loaf pan.

4. In a mixing bowl, combine the flour, baking powder, baking soda, cinnamon, salt, and sugar.

5. In another mixing bowl, whisk together the egg, lemon juice, oil, and vanilla.

6. Pour the egg mixture into the flour mixture and mix until well combined.

7. Fold in the mangoes and dates.

8. Pour the mixture into the loaf pan and place the pan in the grill.

9. Place the loaf pan directly on the grill bake for about 50 to 60 minutes or until a toothpick inserted in the middle of the bread comes out clean.

10. After the baking cycle, remove the loaf pan from the grill and transfer the bread to a wire rack to cool completely.

11. Slice and serve.

Nutrition: Calories: 856 | Total Fat: 41.2g | Saturated Fat: 6.4g Cholesterol: 82mg | Sodium: 641mg Total Carbohydrate 118.9g Dietary Fiber 5.5g Total Sugars: 66.3g | Protein: 10.7g